I0845421

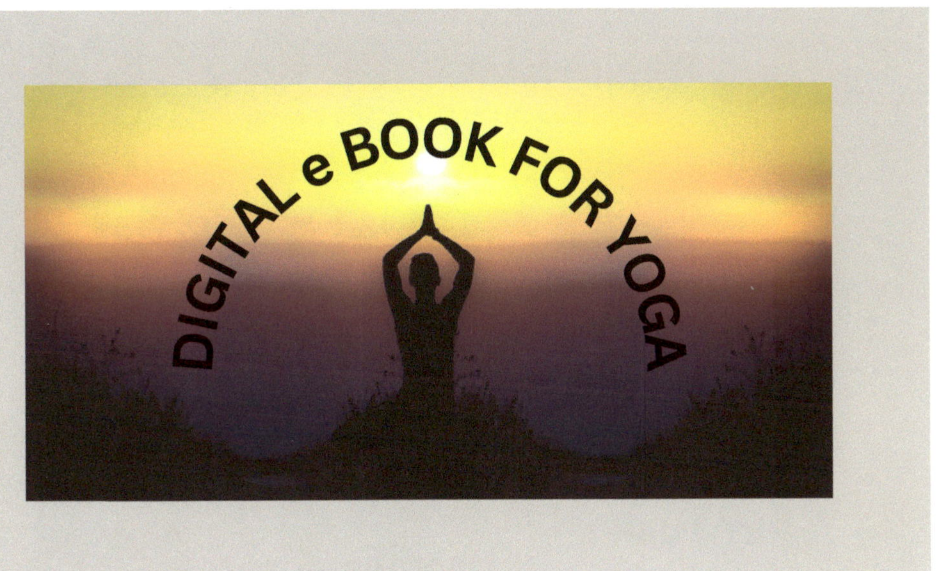

DIGITAL e BOOK FOR YOGA

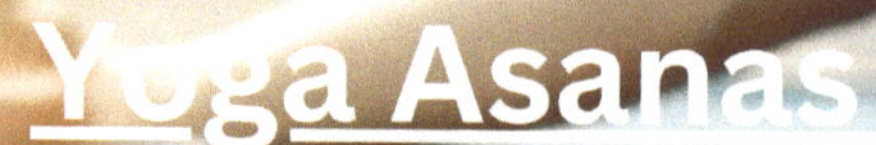

Yoga Asanas
ale the present and Exhale the past
Discipline
Peaceful Life
Relaxing Mind
Happiness
Rich Look
Find your Success Journey

SECTIONS

Yoga - Introduction

Yoga- Exercises

Pranayama

Yoga- for Spinal card

Cooling Pranayama

Effects of Pranayama

Asana- Spinal Card

Asana - Heart

Dhyanam

Mudras

Weightloss

Surya Namaskar

Benefits Of Surya Namaskar

Standing Yoga

Sitting Yoga

Asanas for pancreas

Yoga & Mudra for Pancreas

Yoga for Kidney

Exercises for Kidney

Yoga for Lungs

Digestive System

Exercise for Digestion

Yoga for Neck pain

Yoga for Asthma

Yoga for Back Pain

<u>Yoga</u>

Introduction

Yoga is a Sanskrit word. It is derived from the Sanskrit root word yuki. The word yuki means joining together. Yoga is a practice to relax the mind, body and soul. Yoga is the union of mind, body and soul. Asana means the connection with God in our body through a fixed posture, hence the name Yogasana.

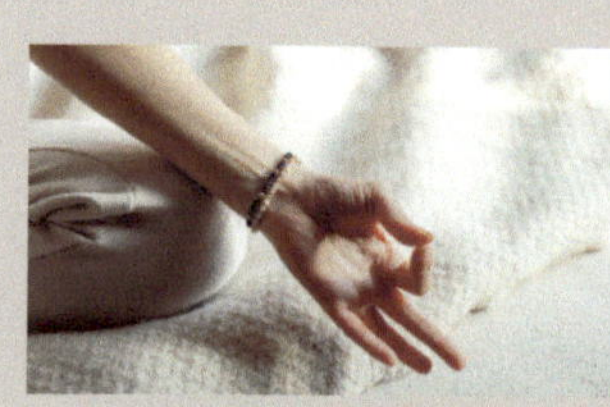

Requirement:
Our mind should be united and practice.
Exercises should be done in a well-ventilated area with a mat spread on the floor.

Nature- Purpose:
The purpose of yoga is physical health and inner peace. Realizing ourself, experiencing the life within ourself.
The same life exists in all. So love everyone with wide love.
Today, everywhere in the world, air traffic accidents are happening. Humanity should grow for this. For this every man should practice the art of yoga. Through this, humanity and good vibes will grow. Body parts are strong and healthy.

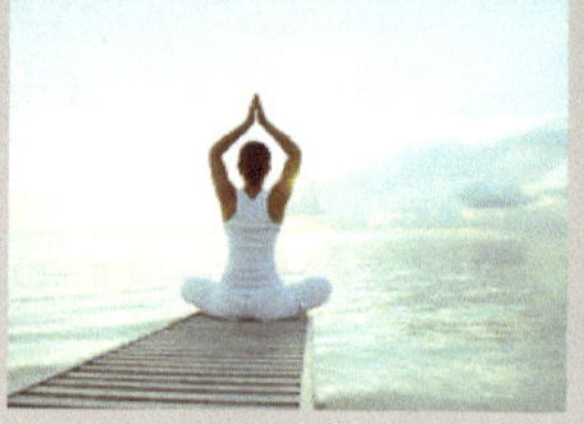

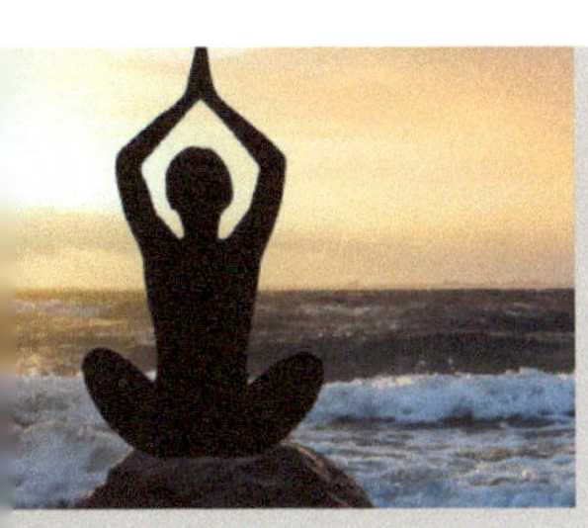

s/heart function well. The
iratory tract is cleansed.
lders are divided and the whole
y flexes. The spine is
gthened.

nervous system on the left / right
of the costal part of the body will
good flexibility. Dehydration is
rolled.

<u>Beginner Yoga Exercises</u>

Proceedure
1. Sit on the rug. Extend both legs straight.
2. Keep the palms close to the hips.
3. Bend the toes of both feet forward and stay in the same position for 10 seconds.
Then bend the toes of both feet backwards and hold for 10 seconds.
Repeat this three times.
Now tilt the right foot slightly and pull the left toes towards the right toe and do the exercise for 10 seconds.
Similarly, relax the left foot and shoot it on the floor and tilt the right foot towards the left leg and hold for 10 seconds.

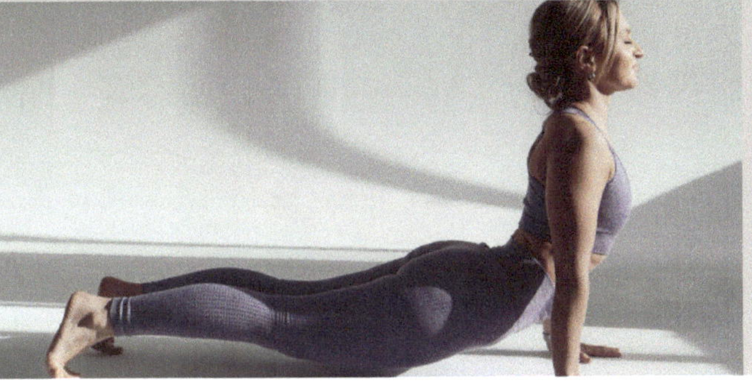

Pranayama

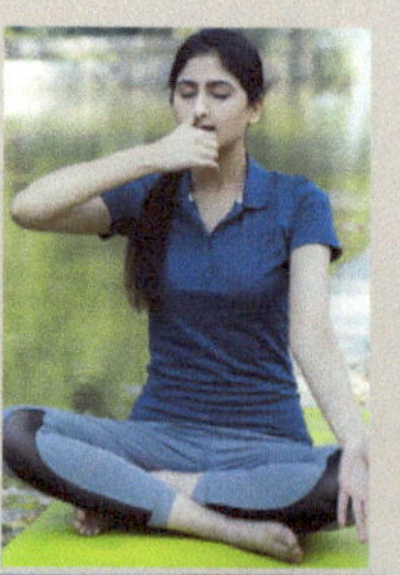

With the right hand close the right nostril with the right thumb and inhale through the left nostril to the count of four. Also close the left nostril with the ring finger and hold the breath for 16 seconds.
Then exhale slowly through the right nostril for a count of 8 and inhale through the right nostril for four seconds and close the right nostril and hold the breath for 16 seconds. Exhale slowly in left nostril for eight counts for eight seconds This is one pranayama.Do ten pranayama morning and evening.

Benefits of Pranayama:

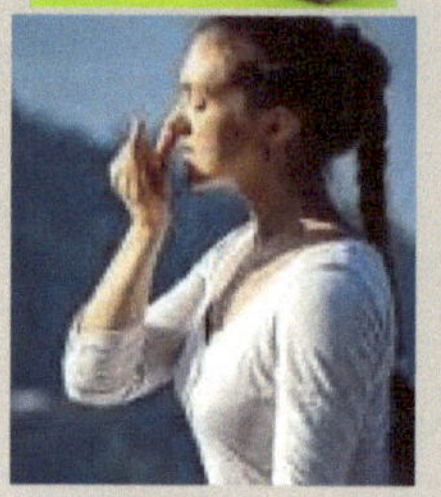

Prana Shakti flows well throughout the body. All the organs get Purana Shakti .All the organs work with energy. Better blood circulation in the body. Heart lungs are strengthened. Better blood flow to the brain. Better brain cells function. Better functioning of the endocrine glands in the body. Live young and energetic. Life expectancy. Increases positive thoughts.Controls diseases like asthma,Sinus headache. Gets immunity. Gains immunity. Relieves constipation. Gets peace of mind Meditation helps too.

Yoga for Spinal card

Functions of the spine

The beauty of a man is his backbone. The most important organ is the spine.In the middle part of the human body, the spine is arranged in a straight line on top of each other.

Cervical vertebrae -7
Thoracic vertebrae - 12
Lumbar vertebrae-5
Coccyx at the base of the spine- 4
Triangular bone of joint under pelvis- 5
Total = 33 bones

Nerves connect the brain and spinal cord. The spinal cord is called the second brain of man. It is this spine that is the point of connection between the brain and the organs of the body.The spinal cord extends from the bulb of the brain down through the bony rings of the spine to the lower back.

Yoga exercises to improve spine

The spine is bent in each asana as the body is bent forward and backward in positions. It strengthens the spine. Those who practice yoga every day will have strong spine.

1. Pirai Asana
2. Padahastasana
3. Pujangasanam
4. Pachimostasana.

<u>Cooling Type Of Pranayama</u>

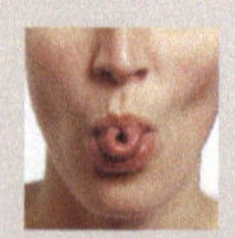

Seethali

Sit up straight on the mat and do Padmasana or mouth breathing slowly and slowly. Close the mouth and exhale through the nose and repeat the same ten times.

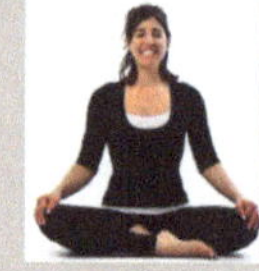

Seethkari

Fold the tongue and breathe in through the mouth, close the mouth and breathe out through the nose, repeat 10 times.

Sakanda

Inhale the air through the rings of and close the mouth and exhale through both nostrils 10 times.

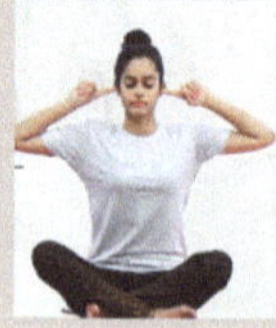

Brahmaari

Breathe in slowly through the nostrils for three seconds, hold for three seconds 15 and then exhale slowly. Then exhale through the nose and throat with a long sound of mu and place your sensation in the throat area and hold your breath for a few seconds and do this ten times.

Effects of Pranayama

Pranayama for students

udents from the age of 7 years can do Nadi
uddhi exercises without holding the breath
d doing so will get many benefits related to
body and mind.
During this period, according to the rapid
physical growth of children, the pituitary
gland begins to secrete the hormone that
stimulates the seasonal growth, thus
affecting the body balance. Due to rapid
owth, the thyroid glands become unable to
nction independently of each other. Due to
this, some children have high physical
evelopment and low mental development
and some students have high mental
velopment and low physical development.

Pranayama for women

Pranayama helps women and according to
the thoughts that arise in a man's heart, the
body becomes radiant, muscular, youthful
and beautiful. If there are no qualities like
anxiety, anger, jealousy, a woman will be
beautiful.
Emotional stress such as anger and anxiety
causes the facial muscles to tighten,
causing facial wrinkles
If girls practice Pranayama during their
school years, they are prevented from
developing traits such as autism, anger and
jealousy.

Spinal Card - Asanas

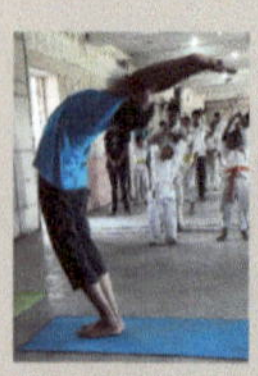

1. Pirai Asana

Stand straight on the mat with both legs together. Keeping both hands on the hips, slowly inhale and bend the back. In that case, you should hold your breath for ten seconds. Then exhale and come straight. Repeat twice.

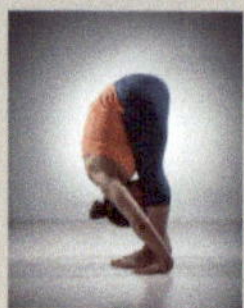

2. Padahastasana

Stand straight with both feet together on the mat. Raise both arms overhead. While exhaling, bend down and extend the big toes touch with fingers. Try to bring the neck part slowly down to touch the big toes. Hold your breath for 10 to 20 seconds.Then slowly come back to normal position. Repeat the same twice.

3. Bujangasanam

Lie down on the mat. Keep both legs together. Place both hands on the side of the heart and slowly arch the back while inhaling. Hold your breath for 10 to 20 seconds. Then slowly exhale and lie down on the floor.

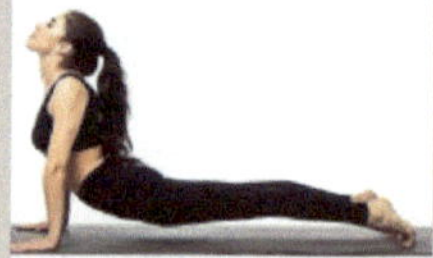

4.Pachimostasana

Sit with both legs extended on the mat. Raise both arms above the head and exhale and touch the toes of both feet. In this case, hold your breath for 10 to 20 seconds. Then slowly extend the arms and return to normal position.

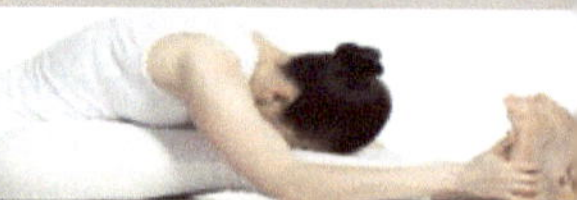

The human body -Heart

Among the internal organs of the human body, the king organ is the heart. Heart Most of the heart is located on the left side of the chest. The weight of the heart is about - 325-400 gms in males. Women have 275-350 grams.

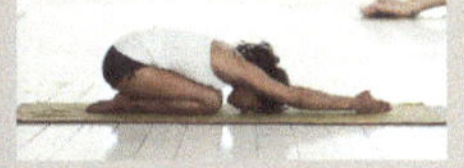

A heart-enhancing yoga matra
1. Usattasana
2. Pujangasanam
3. Nadisuddhi
4. Shunya mudra

3. Nadisuddhi

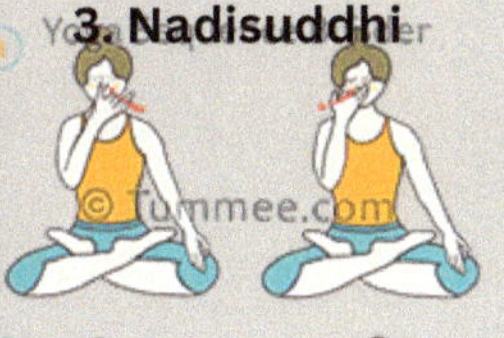

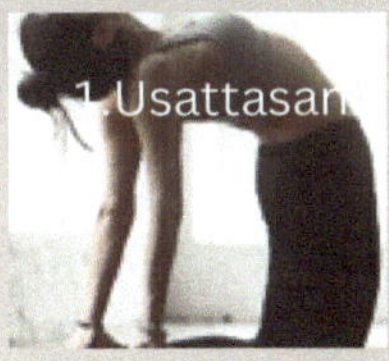

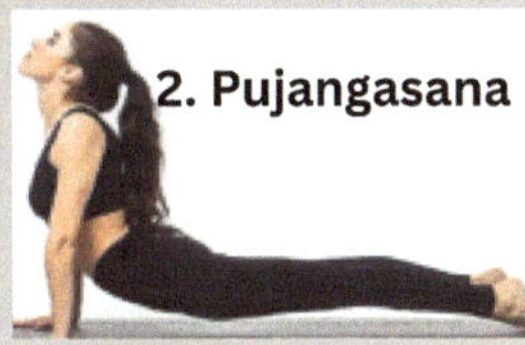

The heart, which is the royal organ , Keep strong by doing simple yoga exercises,

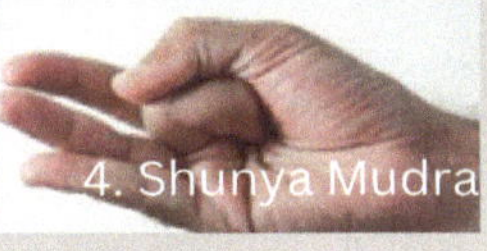

Dhyanam

A man should possess critical thinking abilities
Self-realization begins at the end of a vast item.
The start of focus comes at the conclusion of self-realization.
The conclusion of focus is the start of meditation
The conclusion of mediation marks the start of salvation

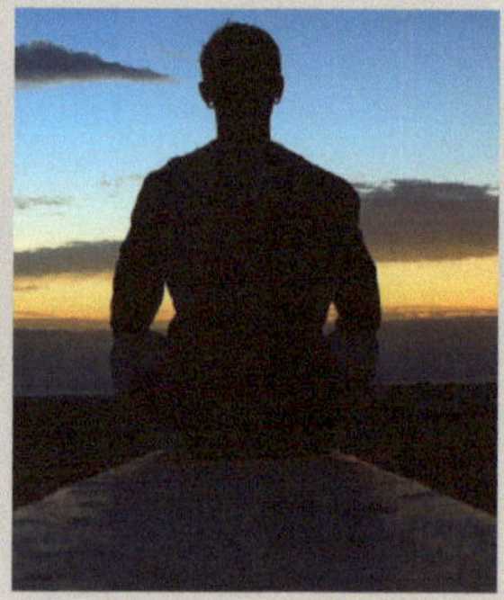

No blood pressure, diabetes, heart pain, anger, greed, jealousy, knowing body, internal organs functioning well, no cancer, if there is cancer, it can be cured by meditation.

Mudhras

The fingers on our body represent this
Panchabhuta philosophy.

Thumb - Fire,
Index Finger - Wind,
Middle Finger - Sky
Ring Finger - Earth ,
Little Finger – Water.

These Mudras should be done with the fingers or
in Padmasana with the hands facing downwards.
The whole mind should be placed under the
pressure of the fingertips.

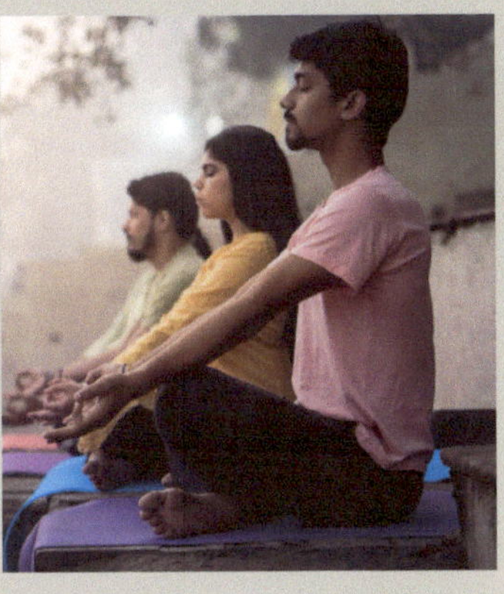

t should be done calmly and with oneness of mind. It can be done both morning and
evening.

Weightloss

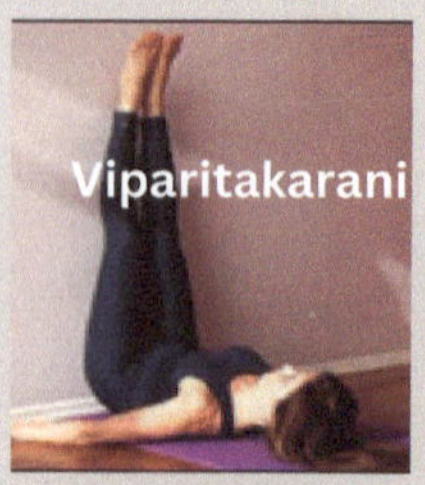

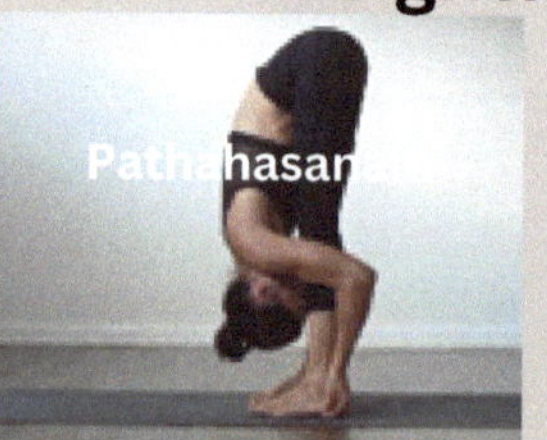

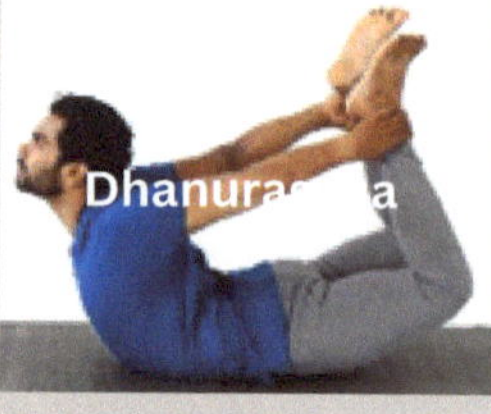

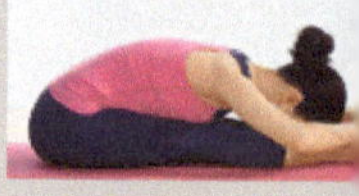

Pachimostasa

Place two pillows one on top of the other on the mat and sit in the center of it and gently lie back with the pillows under the back.
Raise both legs Hold the edge of a pillow with the help of both hands and look at the big toe for five minutes
Then hold the pillow gently with both hands and lie down with the legs down and rest for a minute. Practice this asana in the morning and evening on an empty stomach

Stand straight on the mat, keep both feet together and raise both arms above the head.
Exhale while bending over and touch the big toes and try to move the head to either side of the prop then slowly straighten up and come back to the normal position and do the same twice.

L
ie on your back on a mat, fold both legs and hold the ankles with both hands. While inhaling, slowly raise the head and legs, only the abdomen should touch the floor Hold your breath for 10 to 20 seconds, then exhale and slowly release your hands, lie on the floor, stretch your legs, and rest for ten seconds.

Sit straight on the mat w both hands straight behin head while inhaling bend and touch both toes with help of both hands.
Then hold the normal brea 20 seconds and then rele the hands and come back normal position and repea exercise twice

Surya Namaskar

Thinking of Lord Surya, who protects this world, a yoga practice performed in the morning in the east direction and in the evening in the west direction was designed as a practice of breathing and salutation to Lord Surya with our body. It includes important yoga poses and breathing exercises. This is its highlight.

Mantras

Mantra refines the mind. Mantra removes negative thoughts and provides positive thoughts. The vibrations from the mantra remove the impurities in the blood in the human body and bring light, so in the practice of Surya Namaskar, before starting the practice, the mantra of Lord Surya is chanted with the intention of seeking the grace of Lord Surya and chanting the mantra composed on him and practicing it will have many benefits.

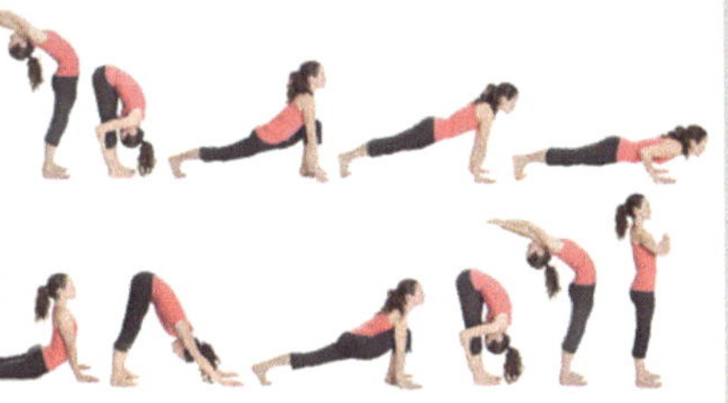

To live harmoniously, it is
necessary to live harmoniously
Praise the glorious Sunday
Praise Surya and praise freedom
Weary praises
Oh or a thousand rays

Benefits of Suryanamaskar

- If Surya Namaskar is done in front of the Sun - diseases related to skin and eyes will be cured.
- As Persian religious priests, Mahans were physicians who practiced healing through sun worship.

An Aryan king who came to Panchalam had a skin disease. He was cured when the Mahans treated him

- Stomach, Lungs, Liver, Spleen, Intestines, Spine gain strength.
- Stimulates respiration, blood flow and digestive system. Nerves are at the center of the brain. This exercise rejuvenates the nerves.
- Focuses the wandering mind.
- A slow general refresher if the body or mind is tired.
- Loses body weight.
- After half an hour before starting this exercise, drink 1 tumbler of water mixed with sugar and the body weight will decrease quickly.
- If women do this exercise regularly, they will produce more milk after conception.
- Corrects menstrual disorders. Prevents week disorders, stomach disorders.

Standing Yogasanas

Utkatasana

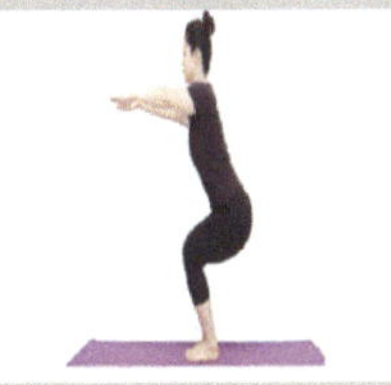

Stand straight with both legs together. Extend both hands one foot apart in front Palms facing the floor. Slowly lower the body slowly as if sitting on a chair. Normal breathing Hold for 30 seconds. Then slowly stand straight. Lower the hands down. Repeat three times.

Benefits
Joints get better joint pain relief Asthma cures shoulder pain Two minutes in this asana gives you all the benefits of walking for two hours.

Tadasana

First stand straight on the mat and share the weight equally on both the legs. Inhale and raise both legs and arms up. Hold the same position for 10 to 20 seconds. Exhale and come back to normal position.

Benefits
Relieve pain in the soles of the feet.is asana helps the students to grow taller

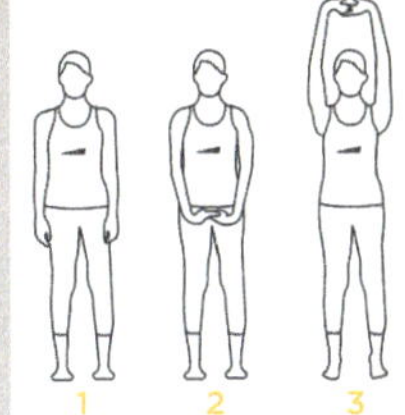

<u>Sitting Yogasanas</u>

Padma Lolasana

First sit in Padmasana and place both hands between the thighs. Lift the body up with the arms crossed and the body should swing on the arms.Then exhale and bring the body to the floor and repeat three times.

<u>Benefits</u>

Strengthened Shoulders. Strengthened colon .Strengthened Pelvis. Strengthened Heart. Strengthened Arms. Strengthened Spine.

Matsyasana

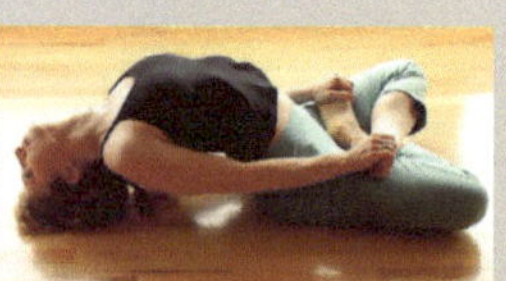

SiSit in Padmasana with the help of both hands bend the head and keep the scalp on the floor and place the hands on both the thighs and remain in normal posture for one minute. Then gently bring the head back to balance with the help of the hands

<u>Benefits</u>

Relieves Asthma. Strengthens Lungs. Relieves Neck Pain. The respiratory tract works well, constipation is relieved, headache is relieved, facial flushing occurs. Get rid of through blood.

Yoga Mudra

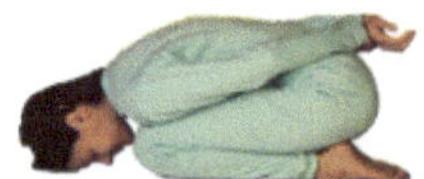

First sit in Padmasana and then alternate both hands and hold the big toes. Then slowly exhale and bend and touch the forehead to the floor and stay for a minute
Then slowly straighten up and come back to normal position and repeat twice.

<u>Benefits</u>

will be lung strength and body beauty will remain intact Liver and spleen will be enriched, tuberculosis will be cured and constipation will be relieved The nerves will get better strength to get rid of the disease by getting rid of throat pain and back pain

Asanas for Pancreas

The pancreas is located in the abdominal region of the human body. It weighs 85 grams.

Functions of the Pancreas

A cellular type of pancreas. Alpha cell, beta cell Beta cell secretes insulin in our body. Insulin regulates blood glucose levels. Excess sugar in the body is stored as glycogen in the liver. Glucogen is converted to glucose in the body whenever needed. Insulin is needed to move this glucose into the cells.

Yoga Exercises to Improve Pancreas

Asana - Dhanurasana, Bhavana Mukkathasana
Mudra - Varuna Mudra, Sumana Mudra

What are the symptoms of high sugar?

Excessive thirst, hunger, vision problems, weight loss, sores in the genitals, sore feet, excessive fatigue, insomnia, leg pain, irritable feet, leg swelling.
People with diabetes can be completely cured by proper yoga practice. Without changing the laws of nature, fasting and eating and doing yoga for 15 minutes every day will prevent the pancreas from becoming dehydrated.

Types of Diabetes:

Juvenile diabetes that affects between 1 and 15 years is called diabetes by the Japanese. From 15 to 30 years of age it is called Pancreatic diabetes. Attacking at 25 is Modi diabetes. Adults above the age of 25 years are susceptible to type 2 diabetes known as Type 2 diabetes.

Yoga & Mudras for Pancreas

Asanas

Dhanurasana

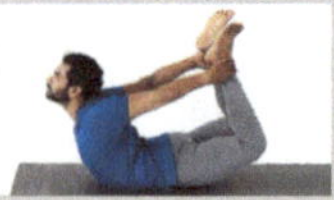

Lie face down on mat and fold both legs. Grasp the ankles of both legs with both hands. Slowly raise your head while inhaling. Raise your legs up. Exhale and hold for 10 to 20 seconds. Exhale and come back to normal. Practice twice in the morning/evening on an empty stomach.

Bhavana Muktasana

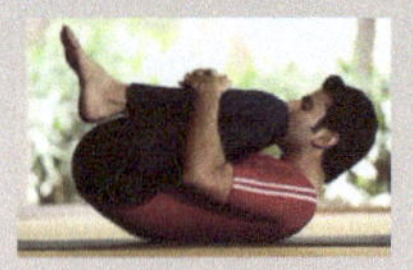

Lie straight on the mat. Keep both legs together. Hold the right ankle joint with both hands while inhaling and slowly touch the knee with the nose. Hold the breath for 10 seconds. Exhale slowly and lie down. Do the same with alternating legs.

Mudras

1.Varuna Mudra

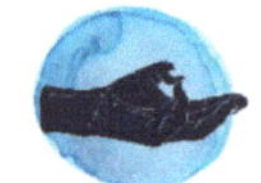

Sit upright on the floor with a mat on the floor. Connect both the little finger and the tip of the thumb. The other three fingers should be pointing towards the floor. Do it with both hands. Stay in this position for 3 to 5 minutes.

2. Sumana Mudra

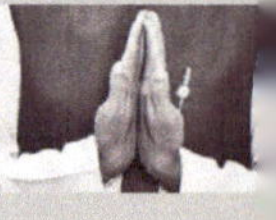

Sit up straight on the mat. Turn both hands backwards so that each finger and nail are joined. Both thumbs should point towards the index finger. Stay like this for 3 to 5 minutes.

<u>Yoga for Kidney</u>

here are about a million urinary nodules in the kidney. These nodules filter urine from the blood and send it to the bladder.
n initial urine output of 125 ml per minute is separated. 150 to 180 milliliters of urine is filtered at this stage
n a day. From the third month of the fetus in the mother's womb until the human being grows and dies, the kidney works without rest.

<u>Symptoms of kidney failure:</u>
enstrual cycle changes, depression, swelling of mbs, fever, loss of appetite, flatulence, cough, phlegm, shortness of breath, muscle spasms, high blood pressure, amnesia.

What causes kidney failure?
Diet, eating without hunger, high blood ressure, taking pain reliever pills, depression, high urea sugar in urine.

Regular diet for good functioning of kidney
Eat when hungry, do simple yogas, nadisuddhi, do simple meditation. If you give proper rest to your body, you should not wake up for too long at night. It is good to eat only healthy food and avoid meat.

Yoga exercises for kidney

Naugasana

Lie straight on the mat. Keep both legs together. Place both hands behind the head. While inhaling, raise your arms and legs until your toes touch your big toes. Do this twice

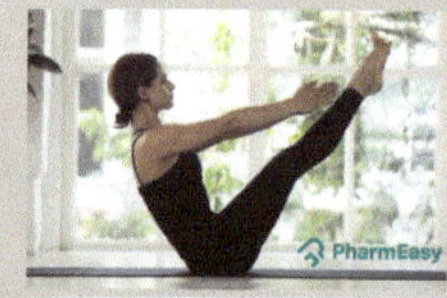

Januseerasana

Sit with both legs extended on the mat. Fold the right leg and place the foot on the left thigh. Raise both arms above the head and while exhaling touch the left big toe and bend down with normal breathing for 10 to 15 seconds. Then stand upright.

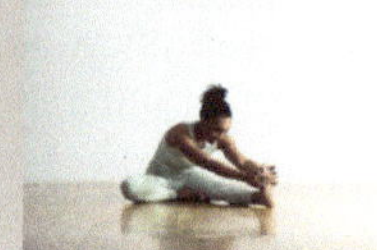

Adi Mudra

Adi mudra may help guide the energy flow to certain parts of the body. It may help improve the flow of oxygen to the body, lower the blood sugar levels and decrease the cortisol levels (stress hormone), thereby perhaps decreasing stress, lowering bad cholesterol and increasing lung capacity.

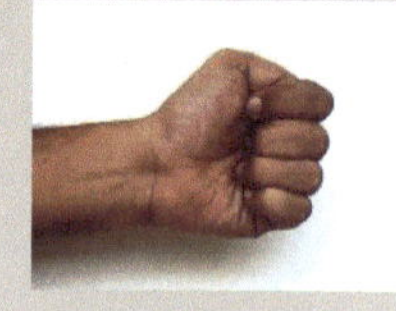

<u>Yoga for Lungs</u>

<u>Functions of Lungs</u>

ir we inhale through the nose passes through the throat through the trachea. At the thoracic region, the trachea divides into two. These are the main respiratory tubes.

n entering the bronchioles, the bronchial tubes twist and branch into several branches. Then from them there are still ler branches - again very small branches that are many branches inside our body that are the lung breathing branches hen air is inhaled, prana gas is taken in, and then the body expels the waste carbon dioxide through lung respiration.

Yoga exercises to improve lung function

Patha Padmasanam

Do Padmasana. Interlace the hands and grasp the left big toe with the right hand. In this case, hold the normal breath for 10 to 20 seconds. Then patiently remove both fingers.

Stand straight on the mat
Keep both legs together. Extend both arms one arm apart.
Slowly lower the body as if sitting in a chair.

Utkattasana

Digestive System

Digestion is the main function of the human body. Whatever we get, we put it in our mouths whether we are hungry or not. And then worry about it? We need to know how it is digested. You have to realize what happens when you eat without being too hungry.

Digestive System – Functions

The alimentary canal looks like a tube. The stomach is like a bag. The stomach is on the left side of the stomach. The esophagus drains from the stomach. The small intestine exits the stomach.

Solution: Apply only when hungry. Conscious eating. Practicing Yoga Nadisuddhi meditation daily keeps the digestive system functioning well.

Yoga Exercises to Improve Digestion

Vajrasana

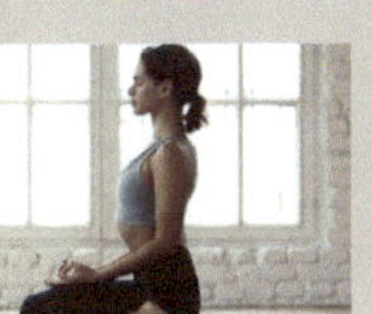

Sit on the rug. Fold each leg and sit with both heels kicked up.
Sit upright with both hands resting on the knees. Close your eyes and inhale very slowly and exhale very slowly. Stay in this position for 2 minutes.

Pachimostasana

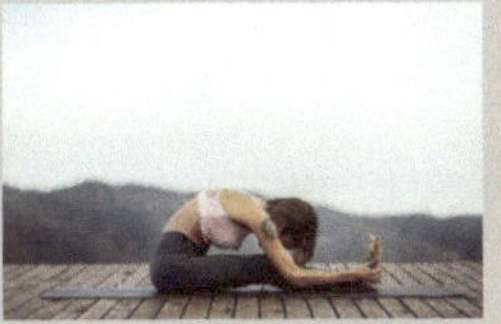

Sit with both legs extended on the mat. Raise both arms above the head and exhale and touch the toes of both feet. In this case, hold your breath for 10 to 20 seconds. Then slowly extend the arms and return to normal position.

Vayu Mudra

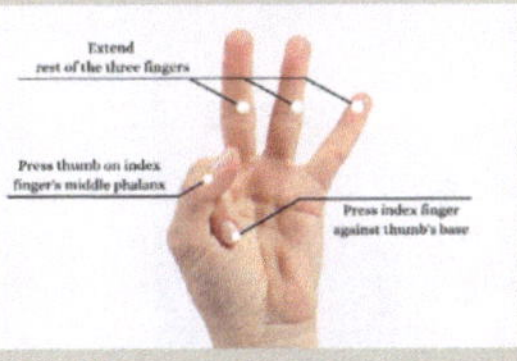

Sit upright on the mat. Fold the index finger and place the thumb on top and apply slight pressure. Do it with both hands. Stay for 2 minutes with normal breathing.

Yoga to get rid of neck pain

Neck pain occurs when there is damage to the flow of energy in the lungs and heart. If there is nasal *congest* *and sinuses in the body, there will be neck pain*

First practice
Sit up straight.
Keep the spine straight.
Inhale slowly and exhale very slowly. Do this ten times.
Now while inhaling, bend both the hands above the head along with the ears.
Inhale slowly through both nostrils and exhale very slowly. Stay for twenty seconds.
Do the same three to five times patiently.

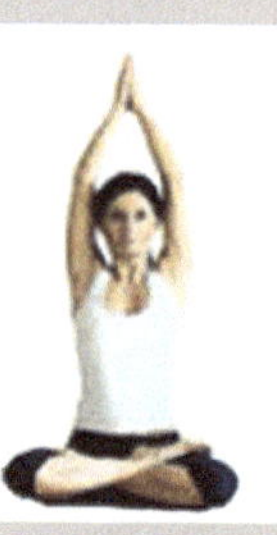

Second exercise
Sit up straight.
Place hands on hips.
Just turn your head slowly to right, back, left, front.
First, start from the right side and make one round, then start from the left side and make one round.
Repeat this exercise twice on each side.

<u>General note:</u>
People with neck pain should not sleep on a very large pillow. Use a very small pillow. You can even fold a pie
into four and keep it on your head.

<u>Yoga for Asthma</u>

Prayer meditation is the first foundation we lay for asthma relief.
Nadi Shuddhi and Pranayama Simple Yoga Asanas can cure countless people suffering from Asthma.

Viparita karani

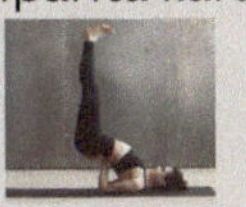

...tack three pillows on the partition in front of ...e pillow. Sit between the tip of the front and ...e center of the seat. Slowly bend back and lie ...down with your hands on the floor and place your scalp on the mat.
...aise both legs together and bring your legs to ...0 degrees so that your shoulders are on the ...at. Place the hands casually by the side of the pillow and breathe normally for two to five minutes
...ng my feet down and put them on the floor to ...ake a break. First the trainees should do this ...th the help of a teacher. After three months of ...ontinuous practice, you can do this asana for 10 minutes

Benefits
...xcellent asana for asthma, relieves headache, reduces body weight and belly.

Machasana

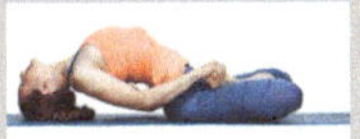

Since machan is doing sarvangasana, you should do saman machasana as an alternative to it.

Sit in Padmasana with the help of both hands bend the head and keep the scalp on the floor and place the hands on both the thighs and remain in normal posture for one minute. Then gently balance the head with the helper in the hands.

Benefits
Asthma is cured Lungs are strengthened Neck pain is relieved.Respiratory system works well. Constipation Relieves.Headache Relieves. Facial Flushing Relieves.

Piraiyasana

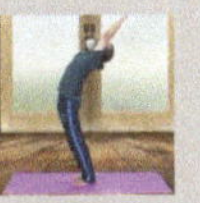

First stand straight on the mat with both legs together put both hands on the hips and inhale slowly bend back.
Exhale for 15 seconds and repeat three times while standing up straight.

Benefits
Strengthens Lungs. Heart Improves. Asthma Relieves. Spinal Cord Relieves. Congestion Sinus Relieves. Back Pain Relieves.

Dhanurasana

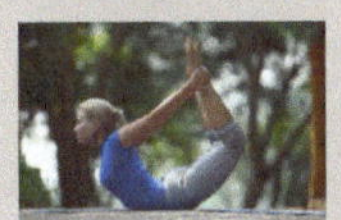

First lie on the mat on your back, fold both legs and hold the ankles of the legs with both hands.
Now bend the legs at the ankles and the back well behind. Inhale and hold the position for 20 seconds and then exhale and come back to the normal position. Repeat three times.

Benefits
Cleanses the body. Removes diabetes. Removes constipation. Reduces excess belly fat. Removes menstrual related ailments for women. Strengthens lungs. Removes asthma.

<u>Yoga for Back Pain</u>

The most beautiful thing in a human being is the backbone. If someone helps us in the progress of our life, we usually say that he is the backbone of my life. Man alone has acquired the position of sleeping with his spine flat on the ground.

Artha Halasana

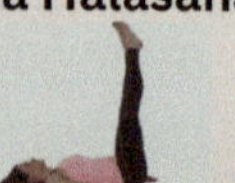

Lie down on the mat and keep both feet together. Keep your hands on the floor and let your fingers touch the floor. Slowly inhale and raise your right leg one foot. Hold your breath and hold the squat for 10 seconds, then slowly exhale and lower your leg to the floor.

Similarly inhale slowly and raise the left leg one step and hold the breath for 10 seconds. Then slowly exhale and lower the leg to the floor and do this three times slowly.

Lie on your back on the mat with your forehead on the floor and place both hands on the sides of your hips with your fingers touching the floor. Now inhale slowly and raise the right leg without folding it, hold the breath and hold it for 10 seconds. Then exhale and lower the leg to the floor.

Then in the same way, inhale the left leg and raise it one step, hold the breath for 10 seconds and let it burn, then slowly exhale and lower the leg to the ground. Do the same three times and raise both legs for 10 seconds.

Artha Salabasana

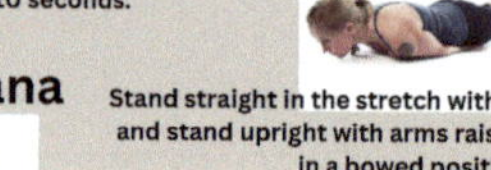

Vrikshasana

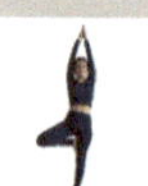

Stand straight on the mat, fold the right leg and place its foot on the left thigh, lift the arms up and bend them for a count of 10, keep a normal breath, then lower the leg and do the same.

Note: For those who practice this first, lean against a wall and raise one leg slowly. Leaning against the wall will be easier at first. After 10 days, after 20 days, you can do it without leaning near the wall.

Tadasana

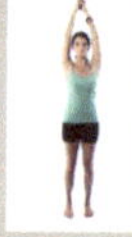

Stand straight in the stretch with both feet together and stand upright with arms raised above the head in a bowed position.

Now inhale and the toes should be on the floor. Slowly raise the body and hold the breath for 10 seconds. Breathe out and bring the arms and legs back to normal position and do this three times slowly without haste

<u>Important Note</u>

People with severe low back pain who have undergone surgery should directly consult a yoga teacher after proper consultation with a doctor

Conclusion

In conclusion, embarking on a journey into the world of yoga through this eBook has the potential to transform your life in profound ways. Through the guidance provided within these pages, you have gained insight into the ancient practices that promote physical health, mental clarity, and spiritual well-being.

By incorporating yoga into your daily routine, you open yourself up to a myriad of benefits that extend far beyond the physical realm. You have the opportunity to cultivate a deeper connection with your body, mind, and spirit, leading to increased self-awareness and inner peace.

Whether you're a seasoned yogi or just beginning your yoga journey, this eBook serves as a valuable resource that you can refer to time and time again. Let it be your companion on your path to health, happiness, and fulfillment.

So, seize this opportunity to embrace the transformative power of yoga and start your journey towards a more balanced, harmonious life today. Namaste.

If you're ready to dive deeper into the world of yoga and unlock its full potential, don't hesitate to purchase this eBook now and begin your transformational journey.

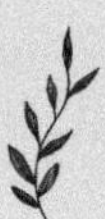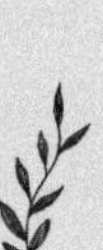

www.ingramcontent.com/pod-product-compliance
Lightning Source LLC
Chambersburg PA
CBHW040320240726
48664CB00006B/1572